Dog Nutrition

Complete Guide On How To Feed Your Dog Age Appropriate Food For Optimal Health

Bruno Michael

Your Free Gift

As a way of thanking you for the purchase, I'd like to offer you a complimentary gift:

- **5 Pillar Life Transformation Checklist:** This short book is about life transformation, presented in bit size pieces for easy implementation. I believe that without such a checklist, you are likely to have a hard time implementing anything in this book and any other thing you set out to do religiously and sticking to it for the long haul. It doesn't matter whether your goals relate to weight loss, relationships, personal finance, investing, personal development, improving communication in your family, your overall health, finances, improving your sex life, resolving issues in your relationship, fighting PMS successfully, investing, running a successful business, traveling etc. With a checklist like this one, you can bet that anything you do will seem a lot easier to implement until the end. Therefore, even if you don't continue reading this book, at least read the one thing that will help you in every other aspect of your life. Grab your copy now by clicking/tapping here or simply enter http://bit.ly/2fantonfreebie into your browser. Your life will never be the same again (if you implement what's in this book), I promise.

PS: I'd like your feedback. If you are happy with this book, please leave a review on Amazon.

Introduction

If you thought the best food you could give a dog, our beloved domestic carnivores is meat, think again. Well, I thought so too; that there is nothing better for a dog other than meat. Therefore, you get it plenty of meat and think that it's getting 5-star food and should be thankful.

Your dog will be full but he or she is not getting all their nutritional needs met from your '5 star diet'. Do not be surprised when its fur does not look as nice or when he starts to develop some funny illnesses because of malnutrition.

A dog, just like a human being, needs a balanced diet for growth and overall health and wellness – which includes being active every day of their life. Yes, a dog is mechanically a carnivore but they are omnivores as well. This means that they can meet their nutritional requirements eating both meat and plants. Now, the question is, 'what exactly do I need to feed my dog, which can be considered a balanced diet?'

This is what this book will teach you. By the time you finish reading this book, you will know what to feed your dog and you will never have to worry about having a malnourished dog.

Table of Contents

Dog Nutrition _____ 1

   Complete Guide On How To Feed Your Dog Age Appropriate Food For Optimal Health _____ 1

Your Free Gift _____ 2

Introduction _____ 3

Chapter 1: Carnivorous Unusual _____ 6

Chapter 2: Dogs' Nutritional Requirements _____ 11

   Factors that determine a dog's nutritional requirements _____ 14

Chapter 3: Nutrients Essential For The Healthy Development Of Your Dog _____ 22

   Protein _____ 22

   Carbohydrates _____ 24

   Fats _____ 25

   Vitamins _____ 27

   Minerals _____ 29

   Water _____ 30

Chapter 4: Feeding Your Dog _____ 33

   Quick facts about feeding any dog _____ 33

Additional Tips _____ 41

Chapter 5: Age Specific Diet _____ 43

The Exclusive Puppy diet _____ 43

Exclusive Adult Dog Diet_____ 55

   Important factors to consider when feeding an adult dog _____ 56

   The Feeding Plan _____ 57

Exclusive Diet For A Senior Dog_____ 61

   Factors to consider when choosing senior dog food _____ 65

Conclusion _____ 67

Do You Like My Book & Approach To Publishing? 68

   1: First, I'd Love It If You Leave a Review of This Book on Amazon. _____ 68

   2: Get Updates When I Publish New Books ___ 68

   3: Grab Some Freebies On Your Way Out; Giving Is Receiving, Right? _____ 68

Chapter 1: Carnivorous Unusual

Why is it that dogs, who are mechanically carnivorous, need anything other than meat?

If we were to classify the dog species in scientific order, it would be in the class of carnivores. It is likely that you studied much about this big group of mammalian animals with a special kind of teeth structure, which allows them to be excellent meat eaters.

However, not all use those teeth for just meat. It is true that some of those animals have an absolute requirement for a meat-based diet. These are called true carnivores. Some good examples of true carnivores include lions and leopards. However, there is another special group, which is a little bit flexible. Despite this group's teeth structure, they can feed on other stuff; they can meet their nutrient needs by feeding on a combination of plant and meat based diet. They are called omnivores and a dog is one very outstanding example, just like humans (the only exemption is that humans do not have those exaggerated carnivorous teeth).

Their tooth and intestinal tract is well adapted

The dog can chew and digest both plant and meat based foods. Therefore, the source of nutrients say for instance protein does not really matter. It can be from beans or beef.

You should not be worried about the source, rather you should worry more about the quality and digestibility of foods – trust me, you do not want a constipated dog in your house.

Let me answer some commonly asked questions about dog nutrition and feeding

Can a dog digest carbohydrates?

Lions may depend on protein for energy, the dog's system may have been designed to operate in a similar way but over time it has evolved to be able to utilize carbohydrates as well. Its digestive system produces enzymes that can digest starches and sugar. Therefore, yes, a dog can digest carbohydrates. They must be included for the sake of a well-balanced diet and for versatility because dogs get bored too from eating the same thing.

Cooked or raw food, which is best?

Lions have no one to cook their food, so they eat it raw ad bloody – this is what they have adapted to. On the other hand, the dog species was domesticated decades ago, and they have someone who cares enough to cook their food. They have adapted to eat like their master, the humans, so they can eat and digest both cooked and raw foods. Actually, they are better placed to digest foods such as complex carbohydrates when cooked.

How many times in a day and when should I feed my dog?

Dogs seem to have an appetite all the time. It can be hard to tell when your dog is hungry or when it is just eating because food is available. This makes it hard to know when or how often you should feed your dog, thus this common question.

Age and sometimes health determines how many times you get to feed your dog. For puppies, you may need to do it at least four times a day. As they grow older but not yet adults, you can let them have 3 meals. An adult dog can eat two times a day.

As for when to feed him/her: The most important thing to note about feeding times is that dogs understand better the language of routine. Therefore, to keep the feeding hassle free, establish a routine. Trust me that you will not have to remember to give them food, they will know it is time to feed and ask for it – by barking, jumping and any other sign they think you understand.

Another good idea is feeding him during family meals. At least he will feel 'included' in family meal times, you are less likely to forget to feed him and it will keep him/her occupied and out of everyone's way so you can all have a peaceful eating experience.

Can I give them bones from the butcher or off my dining plate to chew?

It is true that dogs seem to enjoy chewing bones, which has led us to believe that empty bones are dog food – you are always saving some for him/her. The truth is, dogs do like chewing bones but not all bones are suitable/good for a dog to chew.

There are specific 'bones' that are designed to be chewed by a dog. Those from your plate or the butcher could harm your dog. For instance, chicken bones splitter easily and the sharp little pieces can injure his mouth lining or get logged in his mouth. If they are swallowed, those little fragments will end up in his colon, causing bloody diarrhea or stool. Think about those bigger round bones when you want to give your dog bones. Therefore, if he has to chew any, buy him the special type – they will get the job done while keeping your lovely pet out of harm's way.

How about cat food?

Some people may have told you that they are all domestic animals with almost the same dietary needs so when the dog's food is finished or not available, they can share the cat's. For starters, a dog is in no way related to the cat species. Secondly, they both have different dietary needs because of factors like activity level and weight. A cat requires a higher level of protein and fat to maintain good health.

Your dog may need the same exact nutrients but the difference is in the quantity. By eating cat food, they will end up ingesting more of these nutrients than necessary and gain excess weight – and yes, he will end up becoming a couch potato just like your cat. It can also lead to worse health problems like obesity. While your dog may survive on cat food, but he will never thrive. So, get the dog its own food.

Let us now learn about your dog's nutritional needs.

Chapter 2: Dogs' Nutritional Requirements

What nutrients are essential for the good health of your dog? The answer depends on who or where you ask. Many people do not know what a dog needs. They do not even notice when what they feed the dog has made them sick. There is so much confusion about what they should or should not eat, that is why the answer pertaining to their nutritional needs can vary depending on whom you ask. If dogs have somewhat mimicked their master's diet, why the confusion about their nutritional requirements? Let me explain:

The following explains why many may be confused or misled on what their dog really needs to eat:

Dogs can be made to eat anything

You can make a dog label anything as 'safe for consumption', just by making it available to eat regularly. This is a theory that is confirmed by an experiment done on 3 groups of pups by one Dr. Kuo (1967). To one he fed meat only, to the second he fed vegetables only and the third, he fed a combination of vegetables and meat.

When they grew older, he found that those he fed vegetables ate only vegetables and those he gave meat would not dare eat vegetables. However, to those he gave a combination of vegetables and meat, they became quite flexible dogs; they could eat anything.

There is also another theory that you can teach puppies what to eat by feeding their mother particular foods before they are born. This is because the process of learning what is edible and what is not, starts in the womb when the puppies have a taste of what their mother eats in the amniotic fluid.

Therefore, these theories make us understand that a dog can be taught to eat certain foods or can be switched to even the weirdest of diets from a young age and they will live recognizing it as 'edible' and even pass it on to other generations. This is why no one, not even your best friend is right when they tell you what to give your dog. Just because they exclaim, 'Oh my dog loves peanut butter', it does not mean that you go on and get some for your dog. In terms of suitable nutrition, those kinds of statements are not 'take homes'.

A dog can eat anything. Look at the free roaming village dogs in poor neighborhoods and countries. They have no one to attend to their diet. They go home to eat scraps off their masters' tables and still, they look healthy. Mostly this mess is made of plant-based nutrients (mostly carbs) because meat is considered a luxury. However, they are still able to attend to their protein needs by scavenging on animal matter; carcass, maybe rodents, small birds and lizards. So, yes, a dog can eat anything. They can be best described as adaptive, opportunistic scavenging carnivores. It is up to you to know what to feed it and choose what is best for your dog. Note, what your neighbor feeds their dog and just because the animal loves it does not mean it is the right thing. Mind you, it may get your dog sick.

Dogs won't show sickness; they self-medicate

This is one mammal species notorious for self-medication. A dog will not lie down ill waiting for your medication. If it feels constipated or has stomach upsets because of the crap it ate, it will get rid of the problem before you notice it – especially if you are away or busy. For instance, they find grass perfect for alleviating some 'ill' conditions. A dog will eat grass to help with digestion or ease constipation, to help them vomit, assist with bowel movements or just for nutrition – among other reasons we are not yet aware of.

This is to say that even if you feed your dog crap that is not good for their stomach, they will fix the problem – and it is likely that you will never notice how bad that food you think is good affected it. It is very likely you will give it the same food every day and claim how good you attend to its nutritional needs – and wonder why it does not look as healthy as you expect. Well, there it is, your dog medicates itself when its affected by your poor nutrition choices, and you are confused because you never see them ill and thus you think you are doing the right thing.

So, what determines a dog's nutritional needs.

Factors that determine a dog's nutritional requirements

There is no 'one size suits all' when it come to your pet's nutritional requirement. Dogs are different and they go through different stages all of which determine what they need to eat for good health. So, before you choose their diet, consider the following factors;

Breed

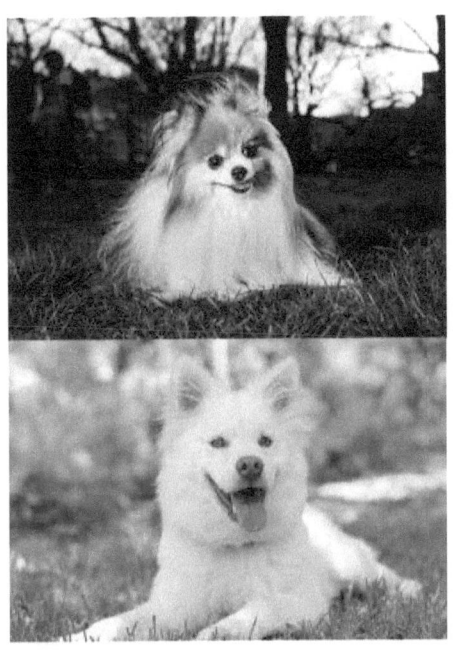

What works for a bulldog will not be good for a Chihuahua or a Bichon Frise. You see a bulldog is heavier than those smaller species. So, how does that matter? Most Dog food companies measure the energy provided in their foods based primarily on the pets' body weight. This in mind, it is important also to note that different breeds have a higher body fat ration to lean mass. Metabolically, fat tissue is considered to be less active compared to muscle (lean mass) thus those 'fatty' and less active breeds have a below average energy requirement compared to their leaner and more active counterparts.

For the above mentioned reasons, it is important to adjust the food and diet, not just by measuring the pet's weight but by considering the breed – because some breeds may weigh heavier because of the muscle while others may weigh heavier because of the fat. The important thing is to get all the nutritional and metabolic information about your dog breed to help you make informed choices.

Age

A puppy and an older dog cannot have similar nutritional needs. It is important to note that dogs go through 3 important life stages; Puppy – adult – Senior, just like human beings go from being an infant to an energy filled youth and adult then to a senior citizen (and retirement). You agree that a toddler cannot eat the same as a super active youth or an older citizen. In the first case, a diet that fosters growth of the mind and body is required while in the last case, food that keeps the now frail bones strong enough not to break with a slight trip is needed.

In the same way, a puppy needs a certain amount of proteins and a special number of calories to be able to transit smoothly and healthily into adulthood. When they get there, their metabolism and nutritional needs change, they need less calories and proteins (to keep them from getting overweight) but more minerals, calcium and fatty acids –

combined with exercise. The old folks need quite a specialized diet. You see, their health has started to deteriorate and they are likely to suffer from illnesses such as urine incontinence, arthritis and conditions that may cause their digestive system to be a little faulty – it comes with age for all animals. Therefore, these animals need fewer calories but high fiber foods (to ease digestion related problems and assist in keeping the kidneys healthy)

So, please consider the age of your dog before you go and feed them something that is going to put them through physical discomfort or deny them the nutrients and energy they need to grow.

Activity level

How active is your dog or rather how active are you? Most of the time, pet's activity level mirrors the lifestyle of their owner. Therefore, if your dog is overweight and sluggish, maybe you are not active too

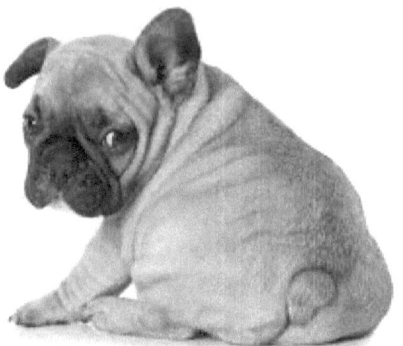

If you have an active dog, it will need energy giving foods.

Working patrol dogs use a lot of calories since they need to be alert to sight, smell and movement on the job even though they may not look like they do much physically.

The hunting (even if they hunt for insects around the compound) herding and performance species spend most of their time expending energy; hence the need for more energy-giving foods.

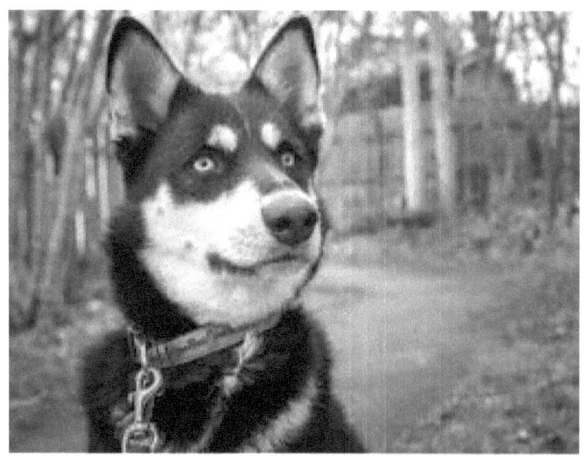

The athlete dog is one that runs or does similar competitive athletic activities; thus, they expend a lot of energy, which means that they will need more energy. The secret is in the normal carnivore diet; you need to understand that carnivores depend on protein and fats for energy. Therefore, the more energy they expend the more energy foods they will require – not the new type on the shelf, boosters or supplements.

So, for active dogs, they will need a lot of energy and repair nutrients. If you give these kinds of food to a dog that cannot get up to chase a ball, it will get obese and lazy and probably die very soon from hypertension or something.

Gender

Are they male or female? Normally male have more muscle mass than their female counterparts who tend to have more fat mass. This means that male dogs require more energy for their extra activity, to build muscle mass and so on.

In gender, we have to consider one very important fact; has the owner chosen to keep his dog intact (maintain its reproductive functions) spay or neuter. A dog that is spayed lacks sexual hormones; no mating or reproducing. Lose of those hormones usually causes the pet to reduce its activity level especially since it has no desire to seek a mate. It will rarely run off to play in the fields or run around the fence sniffing at the neighbor's compound. Whether male or female, it has a higher capacity of gaining weight- but experts say it only happens if they are overfed. Therefore, you have two choices; to make up for the activity by taking it out for runs and walks or playing 'fetch' or reducing its energy intake.

Physiological State

Are they pregnant or lactating? Human beings are usually advised to 'eat for two' when they are in these states, the same applies to your dog. He needs more energy giving foods right now. She also needs to build her strength back and repair whatever body tissues were affected by pregnancy. In this case, you will be going high on protein and fat – and ensure that they have enough water.

Allergies

Be careful to observe your dog to notice how food affects it. If you are giving him the right food for his age, breed, and energy activity and so on and find that instead of having good healthy skin and firm brown stools he has very dull skin, hives or itching coat, there is a problem especially with his diet. He could be sensitive to some components in the food thus the reaction. Note that some allergic reactions could be severe.

It is best to consult a vet whenever you think your dog is sensitive to or has an allergic reaction after feeding him. Let him asses the pet to find out the cause of the problem. You can then work with him to develop a diet that works for your dog.

Preference

Be careful with this one; do not leave a dog to its own devices. It may want a certain type of food all the time, which will not add up to a balanced diet at the end of the day. Thus, you would rather consider more of your preferences (since you are already aware of the right diet for your pet) and train your dog to eat the particular foods you have chosen. Remember, a dog can eat anything. They may not want it at first but if you remain adamant (and not provide likeable substitutes like cookies), they will adapt.

Chapter 3: Nutrients Essential For The Healthy Development Of Your Dog

As mentioned before, there is no one fits all diet for dogs, just like humans beaus each dog is uniquely built and has different needs. However, you need to include some basic nutrients in your dog's diet regardless of their different wants or needs. A balanced diet for your dog will need to contain 6 basic nutrients, which are involved in all the basic functions of the body. Let us discuss them in detail;

Protein

This is a macronutrient, made up of amino acids, the so-called blocks of life.

Its purpose

Protein help the body to build structure; it is essential for building and repairing the walls of vital organs such as the heart and kidneys. It is also important for the development of strong bones and muscles, healthy skin and thick strong hair. Therefore, if you notice that your pet's fur is frail, dull and falling off, you might want to increase their protein intake.

Proteins are also important in the making of hormones (such as the reproductive and growth hormones), important enzymes and antibodies that help the body to function optimally all through. Also, the dog's body can utilize protein to produce energy when carbohydrates and fat used for that are insufficient or unavailable.

It is important to note that protein cannot be stored in their body. If you give them plenty of meat today, do not starve them off protein for a week just because they ate too much days ago. If you do not have a regular source of protein, do not waste it if you have too much today – because the dog will never say no, it will eat it all because it has no awareness of tomorrow. You should know better and spare some even if you have to preserve – in cases of meat. Protein, no matter how much is fed on today will be depleted tomorrow; it is not stored thus your dog requires a constant dietary supply. Therefore, give the dog just enough for the day and more tomorrow and the day after.

Please note

Puppies and pregnant or lactating female require twice as much protein as an adult dog.

Sources of protein

You can get the best protein from animal sources such as eggs, fish and meat. You do not have to give them meat and eggs always, you can also give them quality protein from plant-based sources such as beans, soya and lentils. These are quite affordable and easy to find – and they still get the 'job' done.

Carbohydrates

Carbohydrates are macronutrients that consist of sugars and starches. They are also known to contain indigestible fiber as well – the one notorious for causing constipation.

Their purpose

They are the main source of glucose used to produce the energy that the body runs on. It is important to note that there are unhealthy carbs that are not beneficial for the body – and which only succeed in pumping too much sugar in the dog's body. Did you know that dogs too can develop insulin resistance because of constant high blood sugar levels and get diabetic too, so it's best to steer clear of them.

On the other hand, we have the healthy carbs that contain essential vitamins, antioxidants and minerals that help with various body functions. Other than giving their body energy, they also promote excellent intestinal health and help with digestion – because of the fiber. What's more, they help in the reproductive process.

Ensure you give your dog healthy carbohydrates. When it comes to energy, no need to worry about energy, as dogs can synthesize glucose from protein and use energy from fat. Ask your vet for advice on the best carbohydrates and the right quantities to feed your dog.

Please note

You could exclude carbs if you cannot find healthy ones. However, it is important to note that healthy carbs in the dog's diet is important since the carbohydrates will be utilized longer for energy and spare protein to be used for other more important body functions.

Sources

You can get your pet healthy carbs from legumes, whole grains (those that are gluten free such as oats, barley ....) and Dog-friendly veggies such as carrots, celery, cucumbers etc.

Fats

This is a macronutrient made up of fatty acids. Dietary fats come in three forms; saturated, mono-saturated and poly-saturated.

Their purpose

- ✓ Your lovely pet requires healthy fats to help maintain that healthy skin and keep that fur vibrant and thick.

- ✓ Fats provide a better and more concentrated source of energy than carbs or proteins, because they contain twice as much or more energy.

- ✓ They provide essential fatty acids for growth: omega3s and omega 6, which the dog's body cannot naturally produce. They also help protect internal organs.

- ✓ Fat also helps regulate body temperature, so that it can thrive in changing temperatures and survive even in adverse weather. They are also essential for the optimal health of the nervous system.

<u>Please note</u>

Do not feed your dog excess fat; just because it is good for them does not mean they should eat too much of it. Note that too much fat can cause gastrointestinal issues or pancreatitis.

Sources

You can get healthy fats from fatty animals such as fish; low mercury fish like the salmon and fish oil. These are especially good for Omega 3 fats. Also, there are plant based natural sources such as hempseed and flax seeds.

Vitamins

These are organic compounds required by the dog's body in small quantities to promote better metabolic function. Vitamins do not exist on their own; there is no food that you can give your dog for a certain vitamin say vitamin A. however, they are found in various foods that carry other nutrients.

There are vitamins that are soluble in fat such as Vitamin A, D, E and K. These ones are stored up in the liver and fatty tissues. There are also those which are soluble in water that are not stored up anywhere in the body. It is important to note that a dog's body, just like that of a human being cannot synthesize vitamins from their stores; neither can it produce them on its own. Therefore, they must come from the foods they eat.

Their purpose

✓ They boost the immune system (vitamin A). This helps the disease defense mechanism for the body such that the furry animal does not get sick anyhow – or catch every flu virus that floats by.

- ✓ Vitamin K assists in the clotting of blood, making it unlikely for your dog to bleed excessively when they get little or big cuts or bruises – which at some degree are unavoidable especially for an active dog.

- ✓ Vitamin C and E are antioxidants, helping the cells get rid of toxic substances to promote optimal health of cells which translates to holistic wellness.

- ✓ Then there is Vitamin B12, which is essential for the proper functioning of the nervous system.

Please note

Any home-prepared diet requires vitamin supplementation. However, there are those factory-processed foods which already have these supplements added. They label it 'complete and balanced'. Do not add any vitamin supplements (especially the fat soluble) when preparing the food for your pet as your additional could be an excess and make the food toxic.

Sources

Organ meats and muscle based pieces such as liver, heart or kidneys have a good amount of vitamins

Plant-based sources include pumpkin, dark-leafy greens and legumes.

Minerals

These inorganic compounds play a vital role in ensuring proper metabolic functions in the body. There is no way a dog (or even the human body) can manufacture minerals. It can only extract them from the food it eats.

Minerals include calcium, magnesium, potassium, phosphorus and chloride. These are in the class of macro minerals. There is another class of minerals called micro minerals, which are needed in lesser amounts than their counterparts are. They include iodine, iron, copper, manganese and zinc. Though, it is important to note that both classes are equally important for the body.

Their purpose

Minerals play very important roles that support life. For instance, phosphorus and calcium are responsible for maintaining healthy bones and teeth. Do you realize how much a dog needs their teeth and bones strong? How would they tear into meat or be strong enough to give a good chase?

Also, there is iron, which is needed to aid the process of red blood cells carrying oxygen throughout the body. When a dog has an injury, the mineral called zinc should help with fast wound healing. Also, there are those responsible for ensuring optimal nerve transmission, so that a dog can sense, feel act

– this could save lives you know. Minerals responsible for that include sodium, potassium, magnesium and calcium. Sodium and chloride help regulate fluid balance in the body. Minerals are very important and you cannot afford not to provide your dog with these essential nutrients.

Please note

Puppies need twice as much bone building calcium compared to what an adult dog requires; this is because at that point they are building a 'foundation' for strong bones. It will help with their development to strong adult dogs.

Sources

Almost all foods contain minerals. You only need to know which ones contain which minerals and monitor their quantities and more importantly, ensure quality. For instance, bones are rich in calcium, meat has high phosphorus, fish such as the shellfish are rich in zinc, leafy greens and organ meat have good quantities of iron.

Water

The last and the most important thing that your dog needs is water. Without water, even all those foods we have discussed earlier would not be digested or absorbed in the body. They say a dog can survive without food and proper nutrition;

village dogs in poor neighborhoods are proof. However, without water, the poor animal does not stand a chance.

Its purpose

About 70% of an adult dog's lean mass is made up of water. So, it is safe to say that without water, the dog would not have a body, right? Other than making up the body, there are many other functions but we will mention only but a few important ones. They include:

- It helps in the breaking down (hydrolyzing) of carbohydrates, fat and protein for digestion and production of the much-needed energy.
- 'Washing up' and flushing toxic waste from the body.
- Regulating body temperature
- After food is digested and nutrients extracted, water is responsible for dissolving and transporting those nutrients to cells.
- It also helps in the functioning of the very important nervous system.

Please note:

Human beings are said to need an average of 2 liters of water on a daily basis. Unfortunately, we do not have an exact quantity that fits with all dogs. It is important to note that your pet's water requirements are determined by factors such as weight, health, environment (temperature), the type of food they are fed (dogs that eat high-moisture foods will drink less water than those on dry food) and activeness (activity level).

Another important point to note is that you will never have to measure the amount of water your dog has to drink (there is no counting glasses, thankfully). Dogs are known to self-regulate their water intake to meet their needs. The only thing you can do for them is ensure that they have access to clean and fresh drinking water all through the day.

Chapter 4: Feeding Your Dog

We just put down a long list of nutritional requirements. It's likely that you are wondering how you are going to get all that information and process it into an affordable, simple to make and easy to follow diet that can work for you and your dog. You may also be wondering how to make leafy greens that a dog can eat or how to get them vitamins from pumpkins and all. It would be much easier getting processed foods and pellets – the quick fixes right.

In this chapter, we are going to answer all your feeding questions such as what to feed your dog, in which stage, when and how to prepare it. We are about to learn how to put all those nutritional requirements on a dog's plate. Let's get started;

Quick facts about feeding any dog

Consult your vet

First, before you make any food choices and nutritional decisions, consult your vet. Do this for the sake of being advised on health and nutrition matters from a professional whose studied and dealt with these animals longer – than you maybe.

Your vet will explain your pet's nutritional needs and prescribe a suitable diet considering all factors such as age, medical condition, breed, activity level and so on. This information will help you make informed and better decisions when it comes to food choices for your pet. Also, they can help you create a diet plan.

Note;

Do not swap a visit to the vet for this information for reading food labels in a pet food store. Food manufactures may claim that their food recommendations are guided by advice from renowned vets but what do you know. It may be true but you will find that they rely more on dog stages to guide you; lactating females, puppies and so on. That is quite a broad category to base your decisions on because your dog could be lactating and overweight – the last factor could make a certain food loaded with extra protein and fat to be ruled out.

Such broad categories which food manufacturers are notorious for using are not appropriate to guide your decisions. They may not be able to get into the details but your vet can get to know and access your dog.

The appropriate amount of food to give

You now know that overfeeding results in excess calories and storage of fat in the body, which may eventually lead to obesity, right? This is right for humans and dogs too. As mentioned earlier, a dog can have quite an appetite and if left to its own devices, it will eat more than it needs to – sometimes just to kill boredom.

Did you know that obesity could shorten your pet's life? It plays a major role in the development of killer diseases such as arthritis, diabetes, heart problems and bladder cancer. It is likely that you think that a chubby dog looks cute and feels good to grab but that chubbiness and 'cuteness' can cost you that pet. It is unfortunate that most pets are overweight – and even their owners don't know it.

According to experts, keeping pets lean helps them have a longer and healthier life. This implies that you have to give your dog enough food – calorie restriction will help a great deal. Your goal should be to know your dog's caloric requirement (check with your vet); the amount of calories they require daily to stay healthy and maintain ideal body weight. Make sure that the food you give them in a particular day has the exact calories or will not exceed the appropriate number by more than 10%.

So does this mean that you will have to count calories? You probably will at least in the beginning when you are not familiar with certain foods and their calorie amounts. This is where you have to read food labels carefully and check what foods contain. When you are more acquainted with this information and the measurements, it gets easier – you do not need to count calories unless you are introducing new food.

Raw food

You can give your dog raw food but when it comes to meat, it is not advisable for various reasons. The United States Food and Drug Administration (FDA) advise against it because "feeding raw meat products carries a risk to human and animal health that is significant because of food borne pathogenic bacteria". In simple language, raw meat is not safe because it may harbor bacteria such as salmonella, which cause terrible infections – it can affect both the pet and you for coming into contact with it.

Therefore if you have to give raw meat products;

- Go for human grade meat as it is less likely to be contaminated – and it does not contain harmful preservatives.

- Have a vet nutritionist formulate the diet for you to tell you what is safe and appropriate for age and health of your pet.

- Keep your hygiene standards very high.

Cooked food

Cooked food is great for dogs. However, for meat, you may just have to boil it. This is because sauces such as onion source and other flavors may be good for human consumption but toxic for the dog. Also, avoid cooked bones especially chicken or pork, which soften and can easily splinter.

Commercial Dog Food

Buyers beware! This just sums it up. You cannot entirely believe what is written in those labels. There is no guarantee about the quality of food; it depends on the quality of the ingredients. Cheap ingredients equals to cheap food and a cheap price, therefore if you are buying the lowest priced food, you may as well be buying your dog crap.

Keep in mind that a high price is not a guarantee of quality; companies have been known to overprice cheap ingredients to portray class/quality and attract customers. However, no good thing is sold at a throw away price; so combined with price you can use recommendations and reviews to help you choose the most quality product you can afford. Quality food will cost you but not as much as the visits to the vet if you feed your fury friend cheap low quality food.

It is important to learn the names of ingredients, preservatives and additives that are added to dog food such that you are not confused by the ingredients. Also, it will help if you know which ones have been approved by the regulatory bodies in place, which are safe for your pet.

'All natural' labels do not translate to 'quality whole food'. It may mean that the food is just not overly processed. If you are looking for food free of GMOs, steroids, hormones and antibiotics, you should look for 'organic food' labels.

Commercial food is not as bad as homemade food advocates make it seem. There are manufactures that make quality food, which is convenient in that you do not have to run around looking for all the ingredients required for a balanced diet. The manufacturers do that for you so you can have time to do other things. All you have to do is read labels, be careful with ingredients and amounts of food you give and ensure that the food meets your dog's nutritional needs.

Homemade Dog Food

Just like commercial food, the quality depends on the ingredients used. Most people say homemade food is affordable but what they do is collect scraps from the butcher and leftovers or bad grade food from farmers. The result is poor quality food.

It is important that you choose human grade and good quality ingredients for your dog food. Also, do not just mix things up without nutrition in mind to just fill your dog's tummy. The best thing is to get a prescribed diet from your vet – or have them help you formulate one so you can give your dog what it needs. Homemade is no excuse for sloppiness or bad quality; it should actually be the option that gives the dog the best food given that there is no commercialization.

Fiber

Your dog's food may lack enough fiber. You can get them extra fiber by mixing up their food with cooked pumpkin or raw grated carrots. These should help with digestion and improve bowel movements so that your pet will not be constipated.

Food Allergies

Sometimes your pet may have an allergic reaction to food and since you may be feeding him/her different foods, you may not be able to immediately establish which one caused it. What can you do then?

It is important to understand that allergic reactions are not likely to be inborn. Most of them develop overtime. Therefore, the only way you can figure out what caused an allergic reaction is by doing 'test feeding', which entails feeding the dog different diets and observing him or her. However, this can be challenging because the effects of allergic food can stay in a dog's system for up to 8 weeks.

So, you may have to keep him on a specific test diet for close to 12 weeks before you can try another food – because if you try anything before this time lapses, there may still be the allergy effects which may not be caused by the new food but one that was ingested weeks ago. You may have to do this several times until you figure out which foods cause your fury friend allergies and which ones do not so that you can know what to include and exclude in his diet.

How can you recognize an allery?

Allergic reactions manifest in different forms such as itching, hives on the skin, respiratory difficulties, digestive disturbances and irregular stool. Once you see such signs, consult your vet immediately so that they can evaluate them and make a diagnosis. You will then be advised on the foods to try. Also, make sure that the foods contain minimal or no additives or preservatives.

Additional Tips

- Therapeutic diets; these are special diets used to manage certain health conditions such as obesity, heart and kidney problems. if your pet is diagnosed with a disease, they will need this kind of special diet, which we will discuss more in details later.

- Looking for hypoallergenic foods. Corn could be a good option as it is not a common source of food allergies. Also it is an all natural ingredient containing super nutrients such as proteins, fatty acids and carbohydrates.

- Soy products are good sources of plant based protein – just in case you are vegetarian and do not want your dog to eat meat.

- Beware of semi-moist foods. They have more calories than labeled because they contain excessive sugar, which is used to preserve them. If you are keen on the calorie count, watch out for these foods.

- 'All life stages' labeled food is not all inclusive as manufacturing companies would like you to believe. Apparently, it has been found to contain too much sodium and fat which is not good for adult and senior dogs.

Now that we have established a few do's and don'ts and know more about dog nutrition, let's move forward and find out in detail how to feed dogs in specific stages.

Chapter 5: Age Specific Diet

Let us now break the diet further and focus on specific diet depending on your dog's age.

The Exclusive Puppy diet

At this age, your furry friend is curious and hungry too, most of the time. He's done with mummy's milk and now you need to feed him. He is ready for puppy food and you have to make sure that you start him off right with a good diet and great feeding routine – you know how dogs work well with routines.

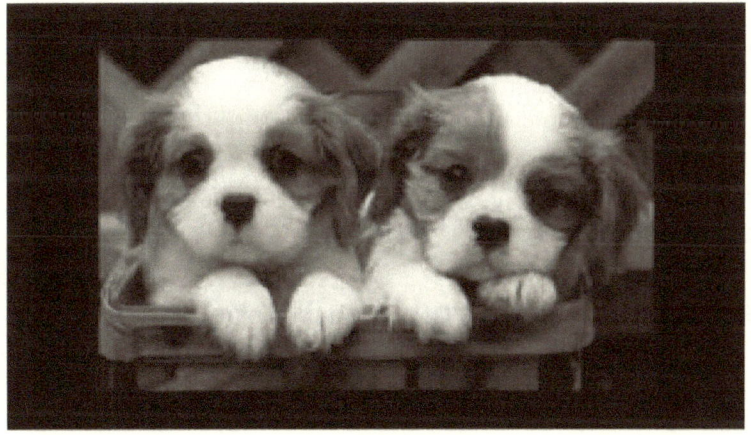

Puppies are the 'raw material' for that adorable, healthy and strong dog you are looking forward to have. This is the time you need to 'build' him from the ground up to be that dog. Proper nutrition and a well balanced diet right from his first meal is what will help build him, therefore you cannot afford to blunder.

Proper nutrition will help build strong bones and teeth, provide energy needed for the hyper activeness associated with puppies (you know how like little kids they find everything fascinating and want to tag and pull even a sock) and the learning you will take him through (you have plenty of tricks to teach him am sure). Also, he needs to build muscle to help with all that running and jumping.

Can you feed your puppy the same diet as your adult dogs? No. They have different nutritional needs; puppies are building their bones, muscle and developing organs while adults are maintaining their bodies. For these reasons, your puppy needs extra nutrients.

The big question: what exactly do you feed your puppy? What is appropriate and healthy? Let's learn below;

Introducing and feeding them solid food

A puppy suckles its mother at birth and can be supplemented with other fluids such as cow milk.

Most puppies of all breed types are ready for weaning by their sixth week. However, in special cases where their mother is not producing enough milk or when they are not able to satisfy their calorie requirement, they can be weaned at four weeks.

Do not be surprised when they do not eat dry corn at 6 six weeks. You need to moisten your puppies' food until it feels spongy, at least until they are about 8 weeks old. There is an exemption for small breed dogs who are ready for un-moistened food by 12 or 13 weeks.

Kind of food

Your puppy's food should be high in protein, enriched with minerals, oils and vitamins – nutrients which are essential for growth. We have discussed earlier some of the foods that have these nutrients.

For commercial puppy food

Most manufacturers will go to great lengths to ensure that their puppy food is of quality and supports puppy growth. However, not all of them do that; this is why you should choose food that has been certified by the quality control bodies such as Association of American Feed Control Officials (AAFCO).

It is important to note that when it comes to dog food, you get what you pay for. The certifying bodies only require the manufacturers to meet minimum nutrient standards. There are those who do just that and there are those who go beyond. Cheaper brands tend to be 'just okay' (and low quality) while the premium and more expensive varieties have higher quality ingredients, which are better for aiding development.

Also, try to find breed formulated food, as it is more specific in what nutrients are needed by your puppy. For instance, large breed puppies need food which supports slow and sustained growth so that they can have a chance to develop strong bones and joints to prevent orthopedic problems – when the body gets heavier than their little frail bones can carry . In this case, their food should not overemphasize protein, fat or too many calories.

How much food

Generally, puppies will need a lot of calories to fuel their rapid growth. So, they eat a lot – but check that it's not too much. In dog nutrition, there goes a famous saying, 'check the dog, not the bowl'. In other words, you need not check what you serve your puppy but the puppy himself; his body condition, which translates to weight and appearance. The body condition scoring system (BCS) should help you with this. Here is how it works:

As for appearances, you should be able to feel their ribs but not see them – if you can see them, that puppy is probably underfed. Also, you should be able to see a nice waist just in front of the hips if you lay him down on his side – a round pot bellied tummy means you are headed to obesity.

The weight should remain healthy; your vet and a little research online will inform you about the optimal and healthy weight of a puppy depending on its particular breed.

The last step is to read the guidelines behind the packet of dog food and adjust the amount you feed your puppy depending on the factors (weight and appearance) above.

How often should they eat?

For puppies who need those extra calories, they can be fed up to four times a day. However, most healthy puppies feed at least three times a day. Therefore, 3-4 times a day is quite all right.

However, if for some reason you cannot afford to feed all those times, you can just feed them 2 times. Whichever way, the dog will adapt and stick to the routine. If you are feeding him too many times, you can tell by how the puppy reacts to the food; for instance, like leaving it on the plate and looking uninterested in a meal. For an underfed puppy, you may notice that they are hungrier than normal or gulp their food very fast, then you need to make the duration between meals shorter meaning you will feed him more times. From such observations, you can be able to make adjustments about the number of times you need to feed your puppy.

Quick Tips

- If you get a puppy that's already been weaning, its best to find out which type of food they were feeding on so that you can either continue with the same or help them transition smoothly to another type of food. It will be good and easier on their stomach if you do.

  Do not just switch up foods often or anyhow whenever you feel like or want to try a new product you just saw at the store – with the catchy sales pitches of how they will make your puppy grow strong or whatever. Consistency is very important when it comes to puppies, as their stomach can be very sensitive to food.

  Making food changes should be done gradually. Actually, it should take one to two week to completely introduce new food. This is how you do it; Add small amounts of the new food, for instance let it be 10% of their meal while the rest is still the old food. Over time, increase the percentage of the new food, gradually, until you get to 100%. This will allow them to adjust and make a smooth transition from one food to another to avoid cases of stomach upsets and diarrhea.

- During the food introduction period, you should not simply put some kibble on their plate. Remember that they have just been suckling and are not familiar with this food. However, you can introduce it little by little. For instance, if you are giving them kibble, you can soak it in the water they drink or puppy formula. They will start licking the new food and getting familiar with the taste so that when you actually give them the food as a main dish, it will not be something too new for them.

- Get your furry little friend accustomed to a feeding routine. You can do this if you feed at specific times during the day. Therefore, you should not leave food lying around for him to nibble on every now and then lest he never learns the schedule. The only exemption is for breeds like the Chihuahua, which are prone to having their blood sugar levels drop if they do not eat for a long time.

- By no chance should you ever feed him off your plate or table. We all know how those cute and pleading eyes can melt our hearts and make you give up your piece of chicken. You promise yourself that it is going to be 'only this once' but remember dogs can learn very fast, especially puppies whose senses are out to study and learn their world. By feeding him off your plate/table, you are teaching him to beg for food scraps. He will never be satisfied with his own food and will make it a habit to beg by the table, a bad behavior that you definitely do not want him to have.

Give your puppy just his food, nothing else no matter how much he is begging for it with his cute eyes– or you think he would find it tasty. It might be tempting to let him have a piece of your tasty bacon – we know you love him too much and want to share your goodies. However, you should resist this temptation because you could do him harm even with your good intentions. How, you may wonder?

Remember that your puppy should eat at specific and counted times in a day. I bet you that you have not counted those little foods as part of his meal. Therefore, it is likely that you are exceeding his calorie count. The result is your puppy ending up overweight or even obese.

- Spicy food is not suitable for puppies because they could actually make him sick leading to diarrhea and vomiting.

- You need to up your cleaning game once you start feeding those little furry friends. They are just like kids, clueless about cleanliness, curious, playful and just messy. Expect that they walk through the food and walk around staining your floors. Also, they are learning how to be dog- dogs hide food and these little puppies will hide the food in the house; thus, creating a mess. This is to say that you should be patient and able to endure a mess and committed to cleaning.

- Find a quiet place for your puppy to have their meals. Puppies can be very easily distracted; hence, the importance of having a quiet place where they can have their meals so that they can focus on the task at hand, which is eating

This quiet place should also help keep other bigger pets away from your puppy's food bowl – they can easily scare him away and have his food. Also, if constantly threatened, the puppy may learn to guard his bowl so fiercely that even you cannot come close. This behavior can escalate and became a danger to you and your household – especially little kids.

Note: A quiet place is not something as grand as getting him his own room. It could be a safe empty corner in your kitchen.

- Dogs love to and are easier to manage when they stick to a schedule. You should start to teach him early when still a puppy; that way you will not have a hard time trying to beat bad habits. For this reason, feed him at the same time every day. If you are not around to do it, make sure that you leave someone responsible enough to do so.

Appropriate food suggestions for your puppy

Commercial food

This option is easy because you find readymade food. Some popular foods for puppies are

- 'Puppy food'
- The regular food labeled 'for all life stages'
- Kibble

Homemade food

This will require extra commitment on your part. You need to find the right and high quality ingredients to meet your puppy's nutritional needs. This option will save you money and make sure that your little furry friend eats freshly made food.

To make good food, do not freelance; find recipes for puppy food (there must be plenty online, just Google it). Here are some websites where you can find recipes developed by veterinary nutritionists: BalanceIT.com. Or PetDiets.com.

Balanced homemade puppy food should have:

- Carbs: like potatoes, rice, corn or pasta

- Vegetables: carrots, green beans, peas, leafy greens such as spinach

- Protein: beef, fish, turkey, chicken, pork

- Fat: vegetable oil or salmon fish oil

- Vitamins and minerals: they are present in most foods but it is best to purchase quality supplements just in case the food does not provide adequate vitamins and minerals.

Once you find a recipe to guide you on how to combine those foods, you can prepare the food in bulk (this should save you a lot of time) and portion into containers. The food can be kept frozen for several months or up to five days if you choose to refrigerate.

How about treats?

Treats can be used as a reward especially when training your dog. However, you cannot just give your dog anything that is sweet and assume that it's a treat. Some of that sweet stuff is not good for him.

Treats to avoid

- Chocolate,
- Nuts (macadamia especially),
- Cake (they contain a lot of artificial sweeteners),
- Fruit such as raisins, grapes, avocados

Treats to give

- Fruits such banana or orange
- Vegetables such as carrots
- Meat (excluding ham)

Exclusive Adult Dog Diet

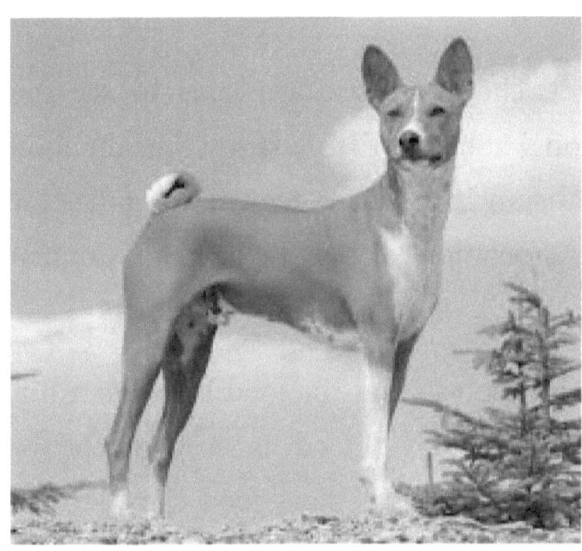

If you have been with your adult dog since he was a puppy, by now you should be well acquainted with their feeding habits, activity level and food preferences. If you just got him, then you can ask the previous caretaker or maybe you can try to study him in the first few months – adults are not as complicated as puppies.

Assuming that you have been with him for a while, you know if he loves snacks and if he likes taking walks, running around or if he just prefers sitting on his mat; this is the kind of information that will help you to choose the best food for him.

Important factors to consider when feeding an adult dog

For commercial food, check the package label to see the statement of nutritional adequacy. It must say that the food meets the nutritional standards set by regulatory bodies for pet food such as Association of American Feed Control Officials (AAFCO).

This statement should also say that the food is fit for 'adult maintenance'. Also 'all life stages food' is okay except for obese or overweight dogs. All life stages food considers all dogs even puppies that as we have discussed earlier need extra nutrients to facilitate growth. An overweight dog cannot have all this extra protein or fat lest his or her health (which is already bad) is threatened.

If you prefer a homemade diet (which many consider cheap) you will need to seek the services of a vet nutritionist to help you design a healthy diet for your dog.

Adult or still a puppy

Your dog size does not make him an adult; some breeds have puppies the size of normal adult dogs. Clearly, you cannot use size or height to determine whether your dog is an adult yet or still a puppy. For instance, there are puppies (for smaller breeds) who grow out of the puppy stage in 7 months while the bigger and giant breeds can take up to 12 months or even more to outgrow that stage – even though for sight assessment they look big enough to be adults.

Therefore, for feeding purposes, you need to know the actual stage your dog is in because giving a puppy adult food won't work; adult/maintenance dog food is made for pets that are past the growth stage. So, how can you confirm that he your dog is now an adult and ready for an adult diet?

When a dog has reached 90% of its expected adult weight (which is determined by its breed and health condition), then it is ready to enter the adults club – at least for feeding purposes. Therefore, you need to do a little research on your dog's breed and when they can be considered to be mature.

The Feeding Plan

Let us now look at an adult dog's feeding plan

The quantity of food

To be honest, a dog will eat all day if there is always food on his plate. Some people think this is 'taking good care' of their dog – by availing something to nibble on all the time. Dogs learn by habit, and they will always want to nibble if you teach them that it is all right to do so. At what risk? They could have a shorter life span when they get obese; you risk losing your furry friend soon.

Give him the right quantity of food to keep him in good health. Taking good care of your little friend is choosing quality over quantity when it comes to food. For right quantities, consider the following;

- Weight: Most food labels will match food quantities with weight range. Check the range that matches. Mostly it is put like this example 5kg – 10kg. If you find that they weigh on the lower side (5) you need to feed the smaller amount.

- Activity level: For lapdogs, you need to reduce up to 10% of the amount recommended for its weight while for active dogs, increase the amount by 20% to 40% as they need more energy.

- Body condition: A lean dog is healthy but sometimes they can be too lean, and this is a health risk just like obesity. We can say that a dog is too lean if its pelvic bone, ribs and vertebrae are visible from a distance. Mostly, this condition is because of underfeeding or an imbalanced diet. On the other hand a dog that is lean enough should not be showing ribs, but you should be able to feel them with your palm and see a waist when you look down on their back (we discussed this in puppies, it is the same way for adult dogs). You can neither feel the ribs of an overweight dog nor see its waist. What are visible are fat deposits on the back.

What can you do?

- Is your dog overweight? Give him less food or choose food that is not too high in calories. You can consult with the vet to come up with a diet plan and calculate the size of portions to help in weight loss. However, it is important to understand that there is a huge difference in giving less food and starving the poor animal. Give him enough (the vet will tell you the 'enough' quantity) lest he loses weight too fast and gets sick.

- Is your dog lean enough? Calculate his caloric requirement, read labels or consult your vet for determination of the right amount of food that is going to keep him that healthy.

- Is your dog too lean? You may need to feed him more calories especially from protein and fat. Your vet will guide you on how long you should do this and how much more you need to feed him.

Please note that it is important to get your vet involved so that you are not guessing around but handling your dog appropriately.

Feeding times in a day

An adult dog has a large enough stomach, unlike the puppy. This means that they eat all their calories in two large meals or even one. However, it is advisable to give him two meals (feed him twice daily) to help him digest the food more easily – and to help control hunger.

Special considerations

An adult dog can reproduce; they can get pregnant. If your dog is expecting little cute puppies soon, you may need to make special considerations in their diet. Check with your vet for guidance.

When they are recovering from an illness or a surgery, their nutritional requirements tends to increase. This is because there is a need for more nutrients for repair, fighting infection and healing.

Exclusive Diet For A Senior Dog

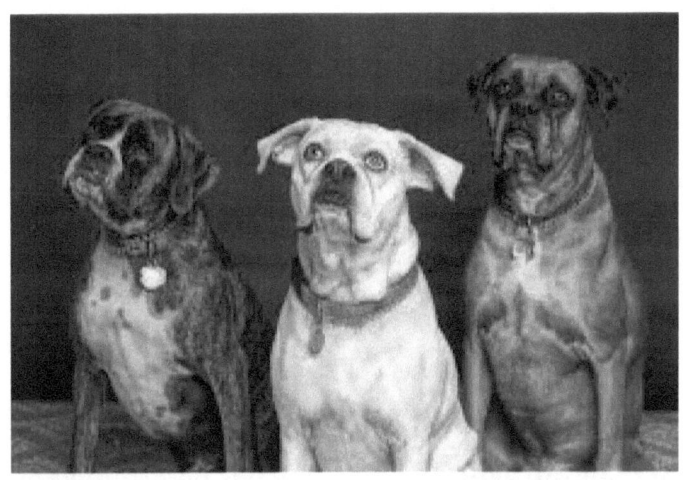

Time has passed and your once little adorable playful pup has gone through adulthood and now they are in their golden years – and maybe not as playful. The dog that could eat anything becomes a little choosy and is not as excited as they used to be. He seems to be practicing a much calmer approach to life – it seems like he knows better now or something.

There is also a major shift in nutritional requirements. He is an adult dog but now, any adult dog food /maintenance food cannot fully satisfy his dietary needs. You will need to make a few changes. Here is how you go about it:

Step 1: Recognize when your dog has reached the senior stage

Has your adult dog transitioned to be a senior? At what age do they make this transition? Experts say that it depends on the breed and their body weight. However, it has been observed that large and giant breeds tend to age faster compared to their smaller counterparts.

The main rule about aging however states that dog are considered to have entered their senior years when they have reached half of their life expectancy – which is determined by breed and size.

The big giant breeds (big dogs) have a shorter life expectancy of 12 to 15 years while the smaller breeds (small dogs) can live upto 15 to 20 years. Therefore, big breeds enter senior stage at around 6 to 7 years while their smaller counterparts get to their golden years at the age of 8 or 9.

Also, watch out for the following signs of aging

- Dental symptoms such as bad breathe and excessive drooling

- Vision or hearing problems – when they take time to respond to your call because they cannot hear you properly

- Lumps on their skin and other issues such as dull fur

When they get older, heading towards the end of the senior period they get to a stage experts call geriatric. Symptoms of this stage are more advanced and include:

- Memory loss (they may not be able to follow their feeding schedule)

- Loss of muscle mass (they get thinner or easily get overweight when overfed)

- Increased urination, which may signify a problem with the kidneys

When you notice the above changes, then your dog is now a senior dog.

Step 2: Discover their special nutritional requirements

A senior dog is not growing and their activity level is not as high as it used to be; therefore, it's only natural that their daily caloric requirements will decrease. In addition, their digestion is not at its peak therefore they need a high-fiber diet to help with matters in the digestive tract and improve gastrointestinal health. Thus, instead of giving dog biscuits as a snack as you previously used to, you may consider vegetable snacks such as carrot and apple slices. You may also need to reconsider high-sodium foods and go for options with lower sodium because dogs at this stage are at risk of suffering from heart diseases.

A senior dog also needs more water owing to the body's inability to maintain water balance. It is therefore important to make sure that they have enough water – their water bowl should never dry up.

Step 3: Find the appropriate food

The 'all stages' labeled foods are okay but in the case of senior dogs, its best that they are not your number one choice. Food made especially for the senior pets should be your go to because they tend to be formulated specially for dogs in this stage.

For instance they have higher quality protein than the standard 'all life stages' and adult foods, which is intended to help the senior pet maintain muscle mass and body weight without putting too much strain on the kidneys – which are not as highly functional as they once was.

Here are other reasons why senior dog food wins over the regular foods:

- Higher digestibility

- Soft texture to address possible dental problems

- Added supplements to strengthen the weakening joints

Factors to consider when choosing senior dog food

Health issues

Below are important things to consider when buying/choosing senior dog food

- Muscle loss: if they have lost their muscle mass, your dog will need more protein foods

- Diminished appetite: If they are eating less than usual, feeding those foods high on vitamins and minerals is a good idea.

- Constipation: choose high fiber diets such as vegetables like green beans and broccoli

Quantity

You may need to exercise potion control as free feeding may cause them to get overweight – since their activity level and metabolism is low.

Dry food or Moist food

They probably start to develop dental issues so dry food may not be as palatable. You can try to moisten their food or feed them raw foods, which tend to have extra moisture.

Ensure you follow the guidelines for feeding your dog to ensure you have a healthy and happy dog.

Conclusion

We have come to the end of the book. Thank you for reading and congratulations for reading until the end.

I truly hope that you have gained great information on dog nutrition to ensure you take good care of your friend and have an amazing time together.

Do You Like My Book & Approach To Publishing?

If you like my writing and style and would love the ease of learning literally everything you can get your hands on from Fantonpublishers.com, I'd really need you to do me either of the following favors.

1: First, I'd Love It If You Leave a Review of This Book on Amazon.

2: Get Updates When I Publish New Books

Visit my Amazon page and subscribe to receive notifications whenever I publish new books.

Check out my dog training books:

Dog Tricks: 15 Tricks You Must Teach Your Dog before Anything Else by Bruno Michael

Dog Separation Anxiety: How To Treat And Prevent Separation Anxiety In Dogs by Bruno Michael

Dog Barking Excessively?: How to Get Your Dog to Stop Barking Excessively

DOG NUTRITION by Bruno Michael

3: Grab Some Freebies On Your Way Out; Giving Is Receiving, Right?

I gave you a complimentary book at the start of the book. If you are still interested, grab it here.

5 Pillar Life Transformation Checklist: http://bit.ly/2fantonfreebie

www.ingramcontent.com/pod-product-compliance
Lightning Source LLC
Chambersburg PA
CBHW030200100526
44592CB00009B/381